This book has been selected
for ... to
bri... ot
ha...ve to ... /.

D0790944

Jenny Craig's
Little Survival Guide

201 tips for managing your weight and your life

Oxmoor
House®

Produced by Time Inc. Ventures Custom Publishing
2100 Lakeshore Drive, Birmingham, Alabama 35209

© 1996 Jenny Craig™ International
445 Marine View Avenue, Suite 300, Del Mar, California 92014

All rights reserved. No part of this book may be reproduced in any
form or by any means without the prior written permission of the
publisher, excepting brief quotes in connection with reviews written
specifically for inclusion in a magazine or newspaper.

Library of Congress Catalog Card Number: 96-70024
ISBN: 0-8487-1552-7

Printed in the U.S.A.
First Printing 1996

Co-created by Jan Strode and Gail Manginelli

Other books you'll enjoy by Jenny Craig:
The Jenny Craig Cookbook
Jenny Craig's What Have You Got To Lose?

Introduction

As I was walking on the beach one morning, I thought about many books I'd seen in the stores on dieting, exercise, and healthful cooking. They all tended to be thick and rather intimidating. Useful if you had a lot of time . . . but not too convenient if you just had a few minutes and were looking for a helpful tip or two.

There really wasn't any type of handy reference guide for the person who wanted to learn more about weight management in an easy, fun way. So I decided to write one. And here it is.

Jenny Craig's Little Survival Guide is a collection of tips and techniques ranging from weight loss and exercise to stress management and cooking.

Some are informational . . . and some are motivational . . . but all are designed to help you reach your weight management goals.

Many of the tips are from our Jenny Craig Weight Management Program. Others come from *The Jenny Craig Cookbook*. We've compiled as many "nuggets" as we could find, because with information comes power — the power to realize your dreams.

Most of you reading this book are probably interested in losing weight. That's great! Because this guide will be a wealth of information and motivation. Think of it as a "companion" that will be right by your side as you go down the path toward a healthier, happier you.

And it really doesn't matter whether you've got 5, 10, 50, or 100 pounds to lose. What does matter is that you've taken the first step to do something about it.

After more than 35 years in the weight management industry, I know what works and what doesn't work. I've found that often the difference between success and failure is just a little motivation and encouragement.

Let this book be *your* source of motivation and encouragement. Refer to it often, especially when you need a little something "extra" to keep yourself going.

I wish you nothing but the best . . . because you deserve it. Here's to your happier, healthier new lifestyle!

Enjoy,

Jenny

*There's no such thing as
an unhealthy food — just unhealthy
portions. Think moderation,
not elimination.*

Skinny up your latte
by ordering it with skim milk;
you'll save 100 calories
and 11 grams of fat!

*Croissants may seem light,
but they're heavy in fat and calories.
Opt for fat-free pastries or muffins,
bagels, or dinner rolls instead.*

Try seasoning with fresh herbs,
lemon juice, stock, wine, or
flavored vinegars instead of adding
butter to your vegetables.

*A cup of ice cream can contain almost
an entire day's allowance of fat grams.
Nonfat yogurt is just as creamy . . .
and much better for you.*

Remember . . . fat free is not calorie free. In fact, reduced-fat peanut butter has the same number of calories as its full-fat version — thanks to its added sugar sources.

Shop the perimeter of the supermarket — the higher fat items tend to be in the center aisles.

As you unpack your groceries, reduce temptation by storing food out of sight.

To get the most nutrients from your fruits and vegetables, choose those with brighter, deeper colors . . . like cantaloupes instead of watermelon, carrots instead of celery, and romaine lettuce instead of iceberg.

*Instant pudding can mean
instant sodium. Just 1 custard cup
contains more than 800 milligrams —
about one-fourth of your
daily sodium allowance.*

Drink a big glass of water
(or two) before cocktail parties where
hors d'oeuvres are served.

Bored or depressed? Don't reach for the refrigerator — reach for a good book or your walking shoes instead!

Invest in a good pair of athletic shoes — they'll make your exercise workouts safer and more fun.

Avocado alert! A medium avocado contains about 300 calories, with a whopping 88% of them from fat.

Put your fork down between bites.

PORTION TIP: 1 teaspoon of margarine is the size of a quarter.

Begin meal preparation before you're very hungry.

Some fruit-flavored bottled waters contain as many as 100 calories per serving. Read the nutrition labels and only buy those with no juices or sweeteners added.

*Buy a 32-ounce sipper bottle,
and carry it with you throughout
the day. It takes just two to get
your recommended 64 ounces or eight
8-ounce glasses of water a day.*

Create a mental picture of what you want. Whenever you start to lose your motivation, pull up that picture in your mind. It'll help keep you on track and moving toward your goals.

Don't have your own 5-pound weights? Start out holding a 16-ounce can of vegetables in each hand and work your way up by gradually increasing the can size.

Give friends and family members
a basket of exotic fruits,
a bowl of potted herbs, or a trio
of homemade flavored vinegars
instead of holiday fudge.

Roasting your Thanksgiving turkey without the stuffing, breast side down, will keep it moist and allow the fat to run off. For a browned top, turn your turkey right side up for the last half hour.

If you can see it, you can be it.

*When dining out, always ask for
your salad dressing on the side. Then
dip your fork into it, so you get just
a little dressing with each bite.*

If you can't avoid "tasting" as you cook, use ¼ teaspoon for each tasting.

Surround yourself with positive, supportive people.

Prepare your grocery list —
and do your shopping —
on a full stomach.

*Replace whole milk with 2% milk;
then 1% milk; then nonfat milk. Make it a
gradual change, and you and your family
won't notice the difference.*

*Move your body at least
15 minutes each day.*

*Start your day with a
well-balanced breakfast.*

*Eat at least two fruit servings a day,
including one high in vitamin C
like oranges, mangoes, or papayas.*

When making flight reservations,
ask the airline about special meal options
like low-fat or vegetarian entrées,
fruit plates, or seafood platters.

Set SMART goals for yourself:
Specific, Motivating, Achievable,
Realistic, and Trackable.
Start with "mini goals" —
they're easier to reach!

*Plan an active vacation: a
walking tour instead of
a bus tour, or a tennis camp
instead of a cruise.*

PORTION TIP: One ounce of cheese is the same size as a Ping-Pong ball.

To lighten up your potato salad, substitute nonfat yogurt for mayonnaise. You'll save about 45 fat grams per ¼ cup.

*When you vacuum, turn on
your portable tape player and clean
in time to your favorite music.*

*Work out in your personal
"comfort zone," so you maximize
results and minimize injuries.*

*Muscle burns calories even
while at rest. To build muscle,
add some light weights or resistance
training to your workouts.*

*Have a small salad, a cup
of soup, or glass of tomato juice
before you leave home. Never go
to a restaurant s-t-a-r-v-i-n-g.*

RECIPE IDEA: For a delicious low-fat, alcohol-free Virgin Mary, mix low-sodium tomato juice with a dash of hot sauce. Serve over ice, and garnish with a celery stick.

You can achieve whatever
you set your mind to.

Things To Do At A Party Besides Eat:

- *Meet new people.*
- *Play a game.*
- *Tell jokes.*
- *Drink lots of water.*
- *Answer the door.*
- *Help the host.*
- *Learn a new dance.*
- *Take pictures.*

Pride is a personal commitment;
it's an attitude which separates
excellence from mediocrity.

*Each time you make a positive choice,
you close the distance between the
way you want to live and the lifestyle
you want to leave behind.*

When traveling for business or pleasure, remember to pack your exercise clothes and swimsuit so you can work out in your hotel's health club.

*On a hot summer day, frozen grapes,
strawberries, or banana slices are
perfect nonfat treats.*

*Only buy canned tuna packed
in water, not oil.*

*If you live in a two-story house,
make trips up the stairs throughout
the day instead of piling things
at the bottom to bring up
on your way to bed.*

Going to a party? Offer to be the designated driver so you can avoid high-calorie alcoholic drinks.

*For extra visibility, always wear
light-colored workout clothes
when walking or jogging.*

Try salsa, flavored mustards, tomato sauce, barbecue sauce, or ketchup instead of mayonnaise-based dressings or sandwich spreads, tartar sauce, or guacamole.

*Substitute nonfat sour cream or
plain nonfat yogurt for
regular sour cream in recipes,
and your family or guests won't
taste the difference.*

Binge-bound? Do your nails instead. You'll keep your hands busy, plus your polish will take a few minutes to dry, which may be just long enough for the urge to go away.

Thin may not happen overnight . . .
but each day will bring you closer
and closer to your goal.

Reward yourself . . . often.
Take a bubble bath, get a massage,
or go shopping — whatever
makes you feel good!

Cook rice and other grains in no-salt-added chicken, beef, or vegetable broth for low-fat flavor.

Jazz up your salad with bitter greens like arugula, radicchio, or chicory.

When using fresh herbs and spices in your recipes, use one tablespoon fresh for every teaspoon dried, and add them at the end of cooking time to preserve freshness. To store, wrap unused portions in damp paper towels, place in plastic bags, and refrigerate.

At restaurants, order first so you're not tempted by what others are ordering.

RECIPE IDEA: For a great side dish, spritz diced or sliced zucchini, red bell peppers, broccoli, carrots, and fresh elephant garlic with olive oil-flavored cooking spray, and roast vegetables at 500° until lightly browned.

*Make the base for low-fat gravy by
adding a few ice cubes to meat
drippings; then remove the fat once
it has hardened on the ice cubes.*

*Ask your waiter to bring out
the basket of bread with
your meal, not before.*

Ask your doctor about iron supplements. You may not be receiving enough iron in your diet, if you eat less than 2,000 calories a day.

*Have you belonged to the
"Clean Plate Club" ever since
you were young? That's okay . . .
as long your plate is full of healthy
choices in moderate portions.*

Alcohol is stored in the body as fat.
Cut down or cut out those
empty calories completely.

Make your home "safe" during the holidays by keeping fattening goodies out of sight (and to a minimum) and donating unwanted food items to charity.

Shake the salt habit — your body gets more than enough sodium from the foods you eat. If you need extra flavor, try lemon juice, pepper, vinegar, low-sodium soy sauce, mustard, or salt-free seasonings.

Use low-fat or all-fruit preserves instead of butter on your bread, or just enjoy the rich taste of the bread alone.

Don't be extreme — be consistent.

Watch your portions when dining out.
Share an entrée with a friend, or ask that
a third or half be "doggie-bagged"
before it's brought out to you.

The next time you slip up, do a "4-Step":

    1 - Forgive yourself.

    2 - Analyze what happened.

    3 - Plan for next time.

    4 - Rehearse your plan.

Fish and seafood are generally lower in fat than almost all meat and poultry. Try them grilled, broiled, poached, baked, or in a salad.

Think of exercising as playing,
not working out.

Success is where preparation
and opportunity cross.

Pack a few nonperishable, low-fat snacks to tide you over while traveling, running errands, or car pooling.

Choose a plain baked potato instead of fries.

Eat three balanced meals and three nutritious snacks daily. Skipping meals slows down your metabolism, which makes it even tougher to lose weight.

*Minimize the nutrients lost while
cooking your vegetables by steaming
or microwaving them instead
of sautéing or boiling.*

If your hotel doesn't have a fitness room, find some stairs. Go up and down as many flights as you can for a terrific workout!

*The old exercise adage,
"No pain, no gain" is wrong and
dangerous. Listen to your body —
it knows what's best for you.*

*Remember that the primary purpose
of a business lunch (or breakfast or
dinner) is to conduct business.*

*Treat yourself to small portions of higher
fat favorites and savor every morsel.*

RECIPE IDEA: Freeze a whole persimmon or kiwifruit for two to three hours. Holding it stem-side down, score the top, peel back the skin, and scoop out the fruit for a frosty sorbet-like treat.

*Eat at least three vegetable servings
a day including one high in vitamin A
like broccoli, carrots, or spinach.*

*One-third of all Americans are overweight.
Don't be one of them.*

Make a list of your achievements.
It'll boost your spirits
and show you just how much
you've accomplished!

PORTION TIP: One-fourth cup of cottage cheese is the same size as a golf ball.

Lean red meat (like cuts from the leg or loin portion) eaten in moderate amounts can be part of a healthy low-fat plan.

Have trouble finding time to exercise?
Break up your routine into
"mini-workouts" and accumulate your
exercise throughout the day!

*Instead of heavy sauces or gravies,
try fruit juices, salsas,
pureed vegetables, broth, wine . . .
or season with herbs and spices.*

*Identify your "High Risk Social Situations"
and come up with strategies on how you
can stay on track. If you always meet
for drinks with friends on Fridays, for
instance, plan to order a diet soda or mineral
water with a twist of lemon or lime.*

Set a healthy example for your children.

Use the 'buddy system' when working out — you'll motivate each other to keep on track.

Cut down on fatty meats like bacon, sausage, and some luncheon meats. If you must — turkey bacon is only 3% fat and 25 calories per slice.

Kick up your heels and go dancing.

*Garnish your low-fat desserts
with fresh raspberries,
lemon curls, or mint sprigs.*

*Drink water during your meal
to help fill you up.*

Need a little something to tide you over?
Try 2 rice cakes, ½ English muffin,
or 3 cups airpopped popcorn. Each
has only about 80 calories.

*Roll away the olives, and serve
an hors d'oeuvre tray with carrot
and celery sticks and green and
red pepper strips instead.*

*Best on baked potatoes: salsa,
butter sprinkles, and fresh chives, or
fat-free Ranch dressing.*

Take the stairs instead of the elevator.

*Looking for a low-fat dessert?
Try angel food cake or fat-free pound cake
topped with seasonal fruit.*

Persistence prevails where all else fails.

When dining out, choose a low-fat appetizer and salad instead of an entrée.

Sauté chicken breasts or vegetables in nonfat cooking spray, low-sodium chicken broth, or wine.

Share your weight-management plans with family and friends for extra support and motivation.

Remember . . . you're not stuck where you are unless you choose to be.

Gardening is a nice way to get in a little exercise . . . plus you can enjoy the results of beautiful flowers or tasty vegetables afterwards.

Add a pasta-pleasin' marinara (tomato-based) sauce instead of alfredo (cheese-based) sauce.

Try a flavored vinegar (like raspberry) on your salad instead of a high-fat salad dressing.

Fanatical about fast food? Try:

- *Grilled meat sandwiches instead of fried*
- *Your burger or sandwich without the cheese*
- *Water, iced tea, diet soda, or skim milk instead of a shake or whole milk*
- *Ketchup or mustard instead of mayonnaise*

Replace "let's do lunch" with
"let's take a walk."

Give yourself a pep talk. After all,
you are your biggest fan!

*Substitute unsweetened applesauce
or nonfat yogurt for oil in boxed
brownie or cake-mix recipes.*

*Be kind to yourself. We all slip up now
and then—we're only human.*

*Weigh yourself once a week —
if that. Your clothes are a
better barometer — they'll be
looser as you get smaller!*

Sweet dips taste best with fresh fruit like apple or pear wedges, grapes, strawberries, pineapple chunks, peach slices, and melon cubes.

*To control portion size,
fix your plate before you
bring it to the table, and leave
serving dishes in the kitchen.*

Drinking eight 8-ounce glasses of water a day isn't as hard as it sounds. Just drink one when you wake up, one when you go to bed, and two with each meal.

Replace breaded or battered meats, fish, poultry, and vegetables with broiled, grilled, or baked ones.

*To keep chicken moist and low fat,
cook it with the skin on; then
remove the skin before serving.*

To add some color to your holiday table, try serving a low-fat dip in scooped-out red and green bell peppers.

Calcium counts! To protect yourself against osteoporosis (bone weakening), have at least three servings of low-fat or nonfat dairy products a day. And consider taking a daily calcium supplement as well.

The next time someone offers you something
you'd rather not eat, try the PRP technique.
Politely acknowledge the offer.
Refuse the offer in a simple, confident manner.
Politely request his/her support in
your healthier lifestyle.

*Walk your dog — Spot or Rover
needs the exercise, too!*

*PORTION TIP: A half-cup of vegetables
is the same size as a tennis ball.*

Chew sugarless gum while cooking, baking, serving food, or while putting leftovers away.

Cross-training helps tone muscles while burning fat. Combine or alternate aerobic activities (like walking or biking) with resistance training (like weight training).

Keep your workout gear in your car or office, so you can exercise at a moment's notice.

Think success!

Believe in yourself.

*Bake your dressing alongside,
instead of in, your turkey. You'll save
fat without sacrificing flavor.*

While eating at home, listen to relaxing music or enjoy conversation instead of watching TV.

Practice meditation or yoga to destress and relax.

Plan ahead, especially when dining out or entertaining. Knowing what you're going to eat beforehand helps you stay on track.

*Think "whole grain" when
choosing breads, pastas, and rice.
Whole grain products are more filling
and much more nutritious.*

*Once you recognize that you're
in charge of your intentions,
you'll realize that you're in charge
of your entire world.*

Try "mini-relaxations" during the day.

- *Take a few deep breaths.*
- *Look out a window.*
- *Pet an animal.*
- *Listen to music.*

- *Stretch.*
- *Close your eyes.*
- *Imagine a peaceful scene.*
- *Enjoy.*

Involve your family in choosing recipes and planning healthy menus.

Fore! Playing 18 holes of golf without a cart requires almost five miles of walking.

*Some people succeed because
they are destined to; most succeed
because they are determined to.*

*Think of water as nature's wine. Serve it
in a crystal glass with a twist of lime.*

When socializing, make friends and family members your focus — not food. Holiday events are "people events" — not "eating events."

*The heavy syrup in canned fruits
adds an extra 120 calories per 1-cup
serving. Opt for fresh fruits or canned
fruits in fruit juice instead.*

RECIPE IDEA: For a creamy white sauce, combine 1 tablespoon cornstarch with ½ cup evaporated skim milk and ½ cup water or broth. Season and cook 1 minute.

*Try low-fat or nonfat salad dressings
as marinades for poultry, fish,
and lean cuts of meat.*

*PORTION TIP: A 4-ounce portion of fish
is the same size as a sunglasses case.*

Don't equate willpower with deprivation. Instead think of willpower as a positive thing — as in "by managing my weight, I will live a healthier lifestyle . . . and I will feel better about myself . . . and I will have more energy for family activities."

Many crackers are loaded with fat and sodium. Look for those with fewer than 3 grams of fat per serving.

Park your car farther from the mall entrance.

All oils aren't created equal.
For cooking, use olive, canola,
peanut, and walnut oils — these
monounsaturated fats may help
lower blood cholesterol levels.

Zesty dips taste great with fat-free crackers or fresh vegetables like broccoli and cauliflower flowerets, carrot and celery sticks, squash slices, and cherry tomatoes.

Try vegetarian at least once a week.
Beans are a protein powerhouse
and a great foundation
for casseroles and burritos.

You're only as old as you feel.

*When cooking or baking, measure
out portions of ingredients; then
return them immediately to the
cupboard or refrigerator.*

Stressed? Try a brisk walk around the block. It'll calm you down and lift your spirits.

The pleasure you get from your life is equal to the 'attitude' you put into it.

Practice good posture. You'll look leaner and feel more confident!

To keep inches off your waist, take inches off your plate. Smaller plates make less food seem like more.

Go for the green — romaine lettuce has six times more vitamin C than iceberg lettuce plus twice as much folic acid.

Add a "dry rub" of mixed herbs and spices to leaner cuts of beef and pork for extra flavor.

During the hectic holiday season, take five quiet minutes each day just for yourself.

Light-meat turkey without the skin is the poultry lowest in fat. Light-meat chicken is also a good choice.

*Help clear the table—remove leftovers
and desserts, and along with them,
the temptation to nibble!*

*Instead of whipped cream, try evaporated
skim milk, chilled and whipped to thicken.*

RECIPE IDEA: Blend ⅓ cup nonfat powdered milk, 1 banana, ½ cup water, and 3 to 5 ice cubes. Add strawberry extract for a delicious low-calorie milk shake!

Fuel your body with "power snacks"
like breads, cereals, and fruits before
or after your workouts.

Don't hibernate in bad weather—go sledding,
ice skating . . . or just throw snowballs!

Plant an herb garden filled with basil, oregano, parsley, chives, and thyme. You'll love the difference fresh herbs make in your recipes.

To see how much weight you've lost, with a piece of string measure the waist of a pair of jeans you wore when you were heavier. Do the same with the jeans you're wearing now and compare the two strings.

Make your nonalcoholic drink look festive with a swizzle stick, umbrella, lemon twist, lime wedge, or celery stick.

The ability to block out the unnecessary puts the goal within reach.

*Put gravy in the refrigerator
so the fat congeals. Then skim
the unwanted fat off the top.*

*Trimming away visible fat from higher
fat red meats can save loads of calories.*

Hard cheeses tend to be high in fat and sodium. Opt for "light" cream cheese or low-fat cottage cheese, mozzarella, or ricotta.

*Fill your buffet table with
fresh flowers, fruits and vegetables,
colored napkins, and other
interesting decorations instead
of fattening chips and dip.*

*For a festive flair, serve your favorite
stew or soup in a hollowed-out
mini-pumpkin, acorn squash,
or Yukon gold potato.*

Don't forget about the salad bar at your supermarket. It's jam-packed with fresh fruits and vegetables—already cut up!

Walk an extra lap around the mall after you've finished your shopping.

More salad bar savvy: Limit or avoid marinated vegetables, croutons, olives, cheeses, sunflower seeds, bacon bits, mayonnaise-based items, and high-fat salad dressings.

If you get the urge to eat between meals,
find something to keep you busy.

- *Call a friend.*
- *Read a magazine.*
- *Write a letter.*
- *Sing.*

Say nice things to yourself and recognize your strengths.

Eat only when sitting at the kitchen or dining room table. A TV tray is not considered a "table."

PORTION TIP: A 3-ounce portion of meat is the same size as a deck of cards, an audiocassette tape, or the palm of a woman's hand.

When cooking or baking, use 2 egg whites or ¼ cup egg substitute instead of a whole egg. RECIPE IDEA: 2 egg whites and 1 yolk instead of 2 whole eggs make great scrambled eggs and omelets with only half the cholesterol!

*If you really want that rich dessert
at a restaurant, order one serving,
forks for everyone, and share.
Or put half on your bread plate, and
ask your waiter to remove the rest.*

*When dining out at a new restaurant,
call ahead and find out which fresh
vegetables, salads, and low-fat entrées
are on the menu. Forewarned is
forearmed — you'll know what to
order before you get there.*

*If you buy butter or margarine,
look for the whipped, lower fat versions
that are usually available in tubs. But use
them sparingly, because they're still
concentrated sources of fat.*

Use preserves and jellies as fat-free sauces or glazes on poultry, meats, vegetables, or fish instead of higher fat gravy and cream sauces.

Commit to the long haul, and make small changes that'll become part of your lifestyle.

With all the hustle and bustle of the holiday season, make exercise the "constant" in your life.

Gingersnaps are the lowest in fat among cookies. Enjoy them in moderation!

And if you like to bake, make sugar cookies or gingerbread men, but don't eat them. Spray them with clear acrylic and use them as decorations or give them away instead.

Degrease meat like a roast by browning it under the broiler rather than on the cooktop. Fats will drip from meat into the roasting pan.

RECIPE IDEA: For tasty oven fries, spray a baking sheet with cooking spray, layer with thinly sliced potatoes, sprinkle with salt-free seasoning, and bake at 350° until golden.

At a buffet, survey the table and decide what you'll have before you get in line. Wait until the line thins; then take only what you had planned. And one trip only.

Toast the New Year with a champagne spritzer — ½ champagne + ½ sparkling water = ½ the calories!

In the end, the only people who fail
are those who don't try.

Ninety-percent of success is
just wanting it.